CONTI

ONE MAN IN FIVE DIES BEFORE HE'S OLD ENOUGH TO RETIRE…

Written and Edited by Jim Pollard • Cartoons by John Byrne • Inspired by Dr Ian Banks, author of the original Man Manual without whom none of this would be possible • Thanks to the advisory board chaired by Dr John Chisholm and all those who helped with the booklet • More credits p35
Fully-revised 4th Edition • Published: Feb 2019 • Revision: Feb 2022.

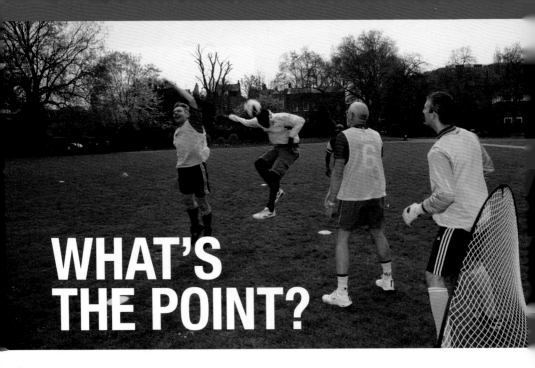

WHAT'S THE POINT?

There are thousands of health books. Most of them make a simple subject complicated. The human body, like the best technology, works out of the box. Understand it, use it sensibly and it'll last for years.

But there's one difference between your body and your new technology or car. If your body breaks down, you can't go out and get a new one (although your partner might) so it makes sense to do some basic maintenance. We can tell you what you need to know in 36 easy-to-read pages.

Scientists reckon that with one careful owner, the male body could run for 100, even 120 years. But it doesn't work out like that.

One man in five will die before he reaches 65, two in five before the age of 75.

Sometimes it's bad luck - an unavoidable accident or something in your genes - but often premature death is down to stuff we can all do something about very easily. We're not talking anything dramatic - just a few little changes that will make life easier and more fun. This booklet will show you how.

SMALL CHANGES - BIG DIFFERENCES

Take the big killers: cancer, heart disease and lung diseases (such as chronic obstructive pulmonary disease - COPD). Most of us will run into at least one of these at some time but there's a lot you can do to delay them, avoid them and even live with them.

There are an estimated 2.5 million people living with cancer in the UK in 2015, rising to 4 million by 2030. As many people now survive the disease as die from it. But it needn't stop there. Nearly 40% of cancer cases could be prevented by lifestyle changes - in raw numbers that means more than 2,500 cancer cases a week are avoidable.

It's similar with heart disease. Deaths from heart diseases are down about 70% since the late 1970s. But again that's because more people are now living with it. The disease remains just as common and indeed hospital admissions are up in recent years. And it's still men who are dying prematurely. Three-quarters of those who die from coronary heart disease under 75 are men.

FAST ACTION - QUICK RECOVERY

So how do you increase your survival chances? Simple: catch it early. That means that if you are worried about anything, get it checked. If you're offered screening or check-ups, go for it.

Reading this booklet and making a few little changes can seriously improve your odds. There is more on all these topics on our website.

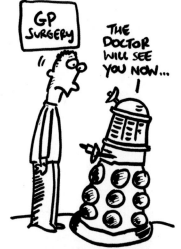

CAN I GET A FREE CHECK-UP?

If you're aged 40-75 in England, ask your GP practice for a free NHS Health Check. It aims to spot early signs of heart disease and stroke, kidney disease, diabetes and dementia and help reduce your risk of these.

The health check was simple - less than twenty minutes.

DO THE MATHS: DO YOU DO THESE?

> NOT SMOKE   > DRINK FEWER THAN 14 UNITS OF ALCOHOL A WEEK

> EAT 5 FRUIT & VEG A DAY > TAKE AT LEAST HALF AN HOUR EXERCISE A DAY

Research shows that doing all four adds about 14 years to your life.

That's time to see your grandchild grow up (or three World Cups!)

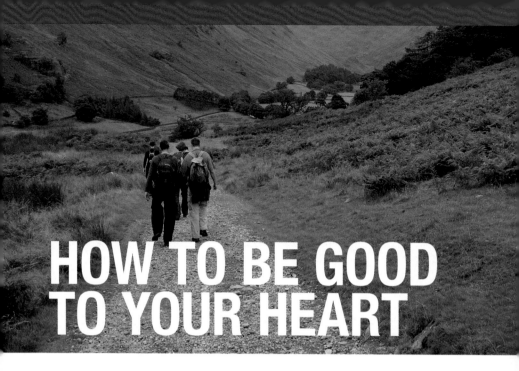

HOW TO BE GOOD TO YOUR HEART

Tune your engine by using the right fuels. The heart needs five things:

> fresh air
> a balanced diet
> a healthy weight
> regular exercise and
> a relaxed attitude.

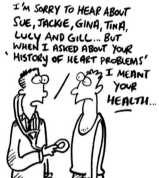

I'M SORRY TO HEAR ABOUT SUE, JACKIE, GINA, TINA, LUCY AND GILL... BUT WHEN I ASKED ABOUT YOUR 'HISTORY OF HEART PROBLEMS' I MEANT YOUR HEALTH...

Heart disease is caused when the arteries that pump your blood get damaged with gunk called plaque. This makes the arteries harden and narrow. The main causes of heart disease are:

> smoking
> high blood pressure
> high cholesterol
> diabetes
> lack of exercise
> being overweight
> family history.

This booklet will help you with all these. For more on the heart-friendly diet, see page 11. For more on exercise and weight, see page 18.

Here's a little incentive to look after your heart:
everything that is good for your heart is good for your penis.

Clear, unblocked arteries mean firm, durable erections. For more on erection problems (an early warning sign for heart disease), see page 22.

I'M A DOCTOR BUT I STILL DIDN'T BELIEVE I WAS HAVING A HEART ATTACK

"

I went to the gym and worked out with three other guys, all in their 20s. I should have thought twice. We did a big routine. The others were sweltering and amazed I'd managed to keep up. So was I.

I had a shower. As I got in the car, the pain began. I was holding the steering wheel with one arm and poking at my chest. As a doctor, I was trying to work out what was wrong. I get indigestion I thought it may be that. Or maybe I'd pulled a muscle or hurt my ribs. When I arrived home, my wife got some anti-inflammatories and called the ambulance. Luckily, it arrived in seven minutes.

I wasn't convinced it was a heart attack until I saw the paramedics' ECG. I couldn't believe it was me.

I had two stents (tiny wire mesh tubes that keep arteries open) within two hours. One of my colleagues did it. I knew the nurse. I was chatting away. It hadn't sunk in. I felt as if I was watching a movie. Alone, after the surgery, I began to realise. You feel vulnerable as a patient. Couldn't even go to the loo. Very sobering.

I was low on all the usual risk factors like blood pressure and cholesterol. Waist is just under 36 inches. But my cardiologist told me half of the world's heart attacks are in the Indian population.

The week-end before I'd been camping with my family on an island. If it had happened there… Well, I figure I've been given a second chance. There's a good chance of depression after a heart attack so I focus on the positives. The problem must have been there for a while and at least it has now been picked up.

It's very humbling. I think it will help me be a better doctor. I've treated people with heart attacks but you feel it's never going to happen to you. Up until now I've always been so well.

Stress can play a big part in inflammation and increase the risk of heart disease. I've always used stress as a motivator. I've enjoyed being calm in stressful situations. I wonder now if doing this regularly has been bad for me. Would I have got this problem with a different lifestyle? I'll never know the answer.

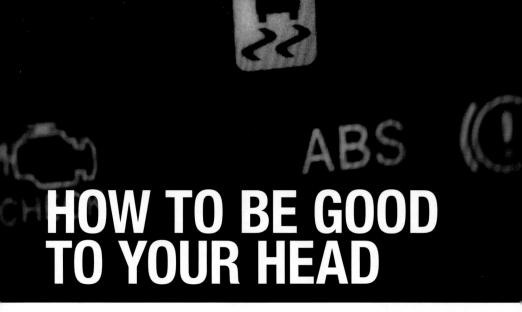

HOW TO BE GOOD TO YOUR HEAD

What's going on between your ears is probably the biggest single factor in your staying healthy. If you feel good, you're more likely to notice when you're ill and to do something about it.

Keep an eye on the main causes of stress: money, work (or lack of it), relationships, drink and drugs, bereavement. Too much stress can:

> damage your immune system and heart

> increase your risk of serious health problems

> reduce life-expectancy

> damage your sex-life.

Get to know what triggers stress and low mood for you.

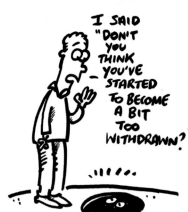

SO HOW DO I BEAT STRESS?

You can beat stress and feel better by:

> eating better - see page 11

> sleeping better - see page 10

> exercising - see page 18

> having fun - singing, dancing and laughing are all proven to boost mood

> not becoming isolated - you don't have to talk about what's stressing you but connecting with other people in even a small way will make you feel better. (Real life contact is better but online is better than nothing.)

> doing something different - volunteering, learning something new

> getting out in the fresh air - especially somewhere green (park, common, countryside)

> learning some relaxation, mindfulness or meditation techniques

> doing something creative

> having sex - cuddles help even if you don't fancy the full works

> finding some time for other things you enjoy.

WHAT ARE THE WARNING SIGNS?

These are the dashboard warning signs. If you spot any of these, ask yourself if they could be early warning signs of stress overload. If they are, do something. The sooner you act, the easier it will be to deal with and the less damage it will cause.

> eating more or less than normal

> mood swings and anger

> low self-esteem

> feeling tense or anxious

> not sleeping properly (or wanting to sleep all the time)

> poor memory or forgetfulness

> excessive drinking and/or drug use

> feeling really tired and lacking in energy

> withdrawing from family and friends

> behaving out of character

> finding it hard to concentrate and struggling at work

> losing interest in things you usually enjoy

> having unusual experiences, like seeing or hearing things that others don't.

There may be physical signs too like headaches, irritable bowel syndrome or aches and pains.

Talking was tough at first but I felt so much better afterwards.

Try to live in the moment. If you're playing with the kids, play with the kids. If you're eating with a friend, eat and chat. Turn off the phone. Don't think about work or whatever's on your mind.

If the warning lights continue to flash, see your GP. Some of these warning lights might have physical causes and, if they don't, there are still many treatments available (and they needn't involve drugs).

But don't ignore the warning lights. Men whose lives are seriously affected by their mental health challenges are not so different from those whose lives are not. Mostly the only difference is treatment and support. So take care of yourself.

There's more on this topic in the Forum's manual Beat Stress, Feel Better.

HOW DO I SLEEP BETTER?

> no screens in the bedroom (includes TV and phones/tablets)

> no stimulants except sex before bed (no coffee, drugs, vigorous exercise, booze etc)

> try some relaxation exercise, yoga or similar

> writing tomorrow's To Do list may clear your head

> reading something light or listening to the radio may relax the mind by distracting it.

THE RUGS DON'T WORK

Male baldness affects most of us sooner or later. Since it's related to testosterone, the only real cure is castration before puberty. Not recommended. The rugs and the drugs are still not great, so better to just relax and remember some of the sexiest men on the planet are bald.

If you're seriously depressed by hair loss, it may be to do with something happening inside your head, not on it.

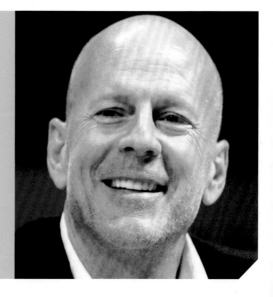

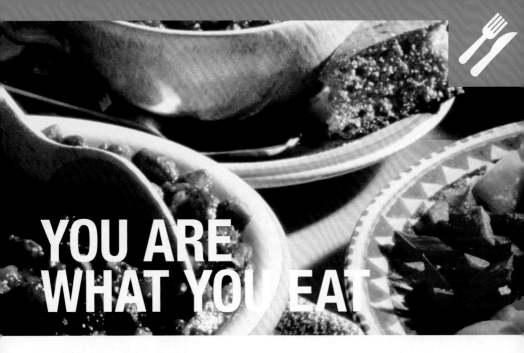

YOU ARE WHAT YOU EAT

Eating better comes with a lot of advantages. It can help you:

> keep a healthy weight

> avoid high blood pressure, high cholesterol, heart disease, stroke, diabetes and some cancers

> exercise better

> work better

> concentrate better

> feel better

> have better sex.

It may even save you money.

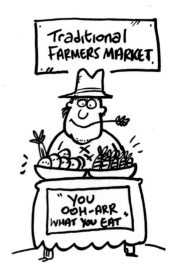

WHAT ARE THE BASICS?

Regular meals help balance swings in your blood sugar levels and reduce swings in mood (grumpiness) and tiredness.

First up, have a decent breakfast. Then, for main meals,

> a bit over a third should be starchy foods like potatoes, pasta and rice. (To boost your fibre, keep the skins on the spuds and go for brown or wholemeal varieties of rice, pasta, quinoa, noodles etc.)

> a bit over a third should be fruit and vegetables - aim for five portions a day

> the rest should be protein (beans, pulses, fish, eggs, meat).

Also make sure you get some dairy (milk, cheese, yoghurt) to keep calcium levels up and bones strong.

> I really enjoy cooking now that I know what I'm doing.

You need a bit of fat but favour unsaturated fats over saturated ones. (Saturated fats are found in meat, dairy, palm and coconut oils.) Avoid trans fats.

Drink plenty of fluids.

Watch out when life changes. When you leave home, move house or job, end or begin relationships, it's easy to forget about what you're eating.

WHAT'S A PORTION OF FRUIT AND VEG

About three heaped tablespoons of veg is a portion; an apple or a banana or similar is a portion of fruit. (Only one portion a day should be juice or a smoothie.)

> There's more on food in the Forum's manual Eat, Drink, Don't Diet.

HOW DO I CURB CRAVINGS?

Eat more slowly so you (and your body) both notice what you're actually eating. This way, you're less likely to eat more than you need and more likely to choose a balanced diet. Go for a walk (even a short one) after your meal - it reduces the rise in blood sugar and fat levels.

If you crave something sweet, distract yourself. Exercise will do this best - a walk or run - as it will also burn off the effects of stress and curb the cravings - but anything that keeps you absorbed will help. If you can't get away, drink water or herbal tea.

Are you really hungry? Often we think we want a snack but we're just thirsty.

BRING ON A SUBSTITUTE

Think about smart substitutions. Fish instead of red meat.
Grilling instead of frying.
Wholegrain instead of white bread, pasta or rice.
Semi-skimmed for full fat.

ANY MORE TIPS?

> Eat mindfully. Sit down and chew each mouthful thoroughly and slowly.

> Don't eat while distracted by TV, phone surfing or reading.

> Choose healthy snacks between meals such as fresh fruit and unsalted nuts.

> Plate smart. You'll get a better idea of what you're eating if you fill your plate just once.

> Go easy on alcohol – it's particularly fattening.

> Keep a food diary - write down everything you eat and drink from when you wake until you go to bed. Accounting for everything that passes your lips helps you make healthier choices and reduce random snacking.

> Read labels. Food nutrition labels help you make healthier choices such as cutting back on salt, sugar and calories.

> Try not to add salt at the table.

> If you choose lower-fat, lower-calorie or lower-sugar versions of foods you eat regularly such as mayonnaise, salad dressings, yoghurt or milk, check labels carefully. Whatever is taken out is usually replaced with something else so low-sugar may be high-fat and low-fat may be high-sugar.

Enjoy all the foods you like but in moderation. If they are full of fat or sugar, simply eat less of them and/or find some healthier options that taste just as good.

COULD I HAVE AN EATING DISORDER?

About a quarter of people with eating disorders are male. Try the SCOFF questionnaire. If you answer 'yes' to two or more of these, you may have an eating disorder. See your GP if you're concerned.

> **Sick**: Do you ever make yourself sick because you feel uncomfortably full?

> **Control**: Do you worry you have lost control over how much you eat?

> **One stone**: Have you recently lost more than one stone (six kilograms) in a three-month period?

> **Fat**: Do you believe yourself to be fat when others say you are too thin?

> **Food**: Would you say that food dominates your life?

WHAT ABOUT DIABETES?

Diabetes causes your blood sugar to become too high. Untreated it can be very dangerous, damaging the heart, eyes, feet and kidneys.

You can reduce your risk of type 2 diabetes - 90% of cases - by following the sort of basic diet and exercise advice you'll find in this booklet. Symptoms of diabetes include:

> feeling unusually thirsty

> feeling unusually tired

> frequent itching around the penis

> cuts or wounds healing more slowly

> peeing more often, especially at night

> loss of muscle

> blurred vision

> unexplained weight-loss.

There's more on diabetes in the Forum's manual **Diabetes For Men.**

IS BOWEL CANCER LINKED TO WHAT I EAT?

Bowel cancer is common with over 40,000 new cases in the UK every year. Most are in people over 60. But younger people are increasingly affected.

You're at increased risk if you have a family history of the disease, smoke, drink alcohol, have a diet high in fat and low in fibre, are overweight and don't exercise. Look out for:

> Bleeding from your back passage and/or blood in stools (your crap)

> A change in bowel habit lasting for 3 weeks or more especially to looser or runny stools

> Unexplained weight loss

> Extreme tiredness for no reason

> A pain or lump in your stomach area.

Ask your GP about bowel cancer screening. Currently, in England, all areas should offer home-testing every two years from 60-74. In some areas, you may be offered a one-off exam at 55. But the government says it intends to lower the screening age to 50. After age 74, screening is on request.

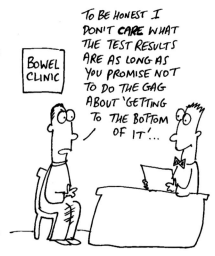

14

I THOUGHT I HAD A BAD BACK
NOT CANCER

"

Looking back, I'd had symptoms for a few years. I put it down to turning 50 and a little bit of irritable bowel syndrome.

The turning point was a holiday with my wife - just the two of us for the first time for ages. She was shocked by how often I was going to the bathroom and I realised just how bad things had got.

I went to the GP as soon as I got back and within three weeks was having chemotherapy. In that short time, I had colonoscopies, blood tests, scans. I've nothing but praise for the NHS – the efficiency and speed, the quality. The nurses are great.

The consultant said the prognosis wasn't good: the cancer had spread from my bowel to liver and lungs. I have an interview before each treatment to see if I'm fit enough for it. So far, I have been.

Nothing prepares you for a cancer diagnosis. But I've learned I'm adaptable. If you had told me I wouldn't have a drink I'd have thought you were mad. You reassess your priorities. Mine are eating and keeping up my weight. (Your weight determines your chemo dose so it's doubly important to keep your strength up.)

I have a nasty thoughts compartment for anything negative. I can't change what's going to happen so there's no point worrying about it. They say the treatment can make you more emotional. But I'm a northern male so I'm not supposed to show my emotions.

I want to stress just one thing: go to your GP. I ignored it and I'm undergoing difficult, expensive treatment for a painful condition. It all might have been avoided had I gone to the GP sooner.

I delayed it because I thought I knew what the problem was. I'd had a bad back for a while which everyone had told me was probably a slipped disc. I was still playing rugby at the age of 56 and didn't want to stop. I knew I'd miss my rugby. And I was right.

Phil died shortly after this piece was first published. His case is one of many that led to the government promising to lower the bowel cancer screening age to 50.

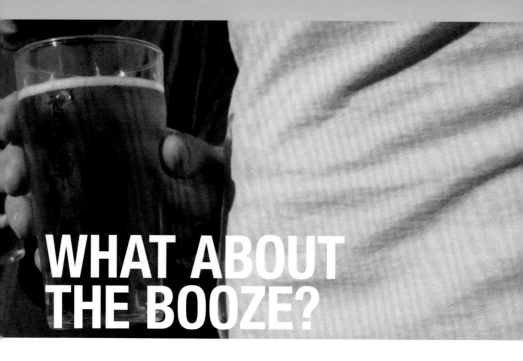

WHAT ABOUT THE BOOZE?

Too much alcohol damages nearly every organ in the body. It can cause heart disease, nerve damage, liver disease, depression, erectile dysfunction, cancer and digestive problems. If you're worried that you're becoming too keen on the drink, ask yourself the 'am I addicted?' questions on page 28.

HOW DO I KEEP AN EYE ON MY DRINKING?

If you want to watch your drinking, here are some trusted ways to do it:

> Drink water - both during the day and to cut appetite before eating and drinking.

> Stop drinking for a week or a month.

> Avoid drinking on at least two nights a week. Increase it to three then four and so on.

> Record each day how much you drink — seeing it in black and white helps.

HERE YOU GO... ALTHOUGH I'M STILL NOT ENTIRELY CONVINCED THAT A SLICE OF LIME IN YOUR VODKA COUNTS TOWARDS YOUR 'FIVE A DAY'...

> If there is a situation in which you always have a drink - for example, after work - try to cut it out.

> When out for the evening, try not to drink more than one drink an hour. Or set yourself a maximum and stick to it. Or both.

> Make your first drink a soft one.

> Reduce the strength of what you're drinking.

> Don't get into rounds.

> Say "No" every so often.

I feel better and more alert since I cut down the booze.

Try a few of these ideas. If you can't do them then you need to stop drinking. If you can't stop drinking, you need to get advice.

The NHS advises men (and women) to drink no more than 14 units a week and to spread that over at least three days. (A pint of 5.2% lager is 3 units.)

HOW QUICKLY DOES THE BODY PROCESS ALCOHOL?

Your liver can process about one unit of alcohol an hour. If you drink any more than that (and the average pint is over 2 units), the alcohol will stay in your system until the liver can process it. That's why if you drink a lot, you can still be unsafe to drive or operate machinery next morning.

There's more on alcohol in the Forum's manual Serious Drinking.

Avoid binge drinking. The NHS defines this as six units or more of alcohol in a single session.

HOW MUCH ALCOHOL IS IN YOUR DRINK?

Large glass of wine (175ml) 15% alcohol	3 units	120-170 calories
Small glass of wine (125ml) 12%	1.5 units	85-120 calories
Bottle of wine (750ml) 12%	9 units	510-720 calories
Pint of beer 5%	3 units	180 calories
Pint of beer 3.5%	2 units	160-170 calories
Single measure of spirits (25ml) 40%	1 unit	60-75 calories

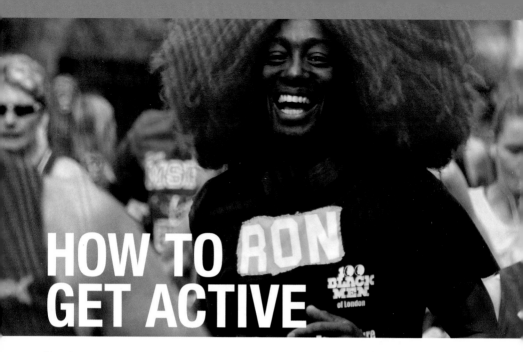

HOW TO GET ACTIVE

Don't underestimate it. If exercise were a drug, we'd all want to take it.
Exercise boosts physical and mental wellbeing and helps you live longer.

Scientists now reckon being inactive is even more of a health risk than being overweight. People who do regular physical activity have a:

> 30% lower risk of depression and of dementia

> 35% lower risk of heart disease and stroke

> 50% lower risk of diabetes and of bowel cancer.

Regular exercisers also have a far lower risk of osteoarthritis and hip fracture.

Best of all, exercise feels good. It boosts feel-good chemicals that raise self-esteem and helps sleep and concentration.

WHAT DOES 'REGULAR PHYSICAL ACTIVITY' MEAN?

To get the full benefit, the NHS reckons you need 150 minutes a week of moderate-intensity aerobic exercise. This means exercise that makes you slightly breathless - fast walking, cycling, jogging, mowing the lawn, swimming, playing sport. The statistics about the benefits of exercise are based on these sorts of exercise levels.

And, if your exercise goal is to lose weight, you probably need to do more than this.

But - and it's a very big but - anything is better than nothing.

Try walking. Walking reduces the risk of heart disease by a third. The further and faster you walk the better but even walking just 5-6 miles a week at a very slow pace (2 miles per hour) will help reduce risk. Little and often is fine. Regular walkers can burn more energy than gym-users.

There are apps and fit-bits to help set targets. Counting steps is a good simple one. Aim for 10,000 steps a day.

Stretching and strengthening muscle are also important. Again, this doesn't have to be vigorous. Yoga is fine. Even very simple exercises such as sit-to-stand, heel raises and marching on the spot can make a big difference when you first start exercising again.

Keep hydrated during and after exercise. Unless you're a pro athlete, water is usually the best bet.

I HAVEN'T GOT TIME.

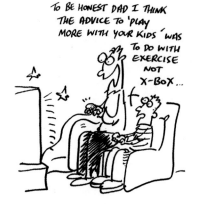

Build exercise into your everyday life:

> get off the bus/train/tram a stop or two early

> park the car and walk

> cycle instead

> use the stairs

> exercise in your lunch-break (even more importantly, always take a lunch-break)

> exercise at home or in the park - you don't need to go to a gym

> play more with your kids

> get into housework and gardening

> walk and talk (on the phone or with colleagues).

Can work help? Some employers have a gym or offer gym membership or cycle-to-work schemes.

Try so-called 'exercise-snacking'. Six five minute walks can be just as effective as one half-hour session.

Combine exercise with your social life by joining a gym, club or team. Increasingly, there are sports opportunities for people of all ages and abilities. But make sure you're fit enough to avoid injury.

I HAVEN'T EXERCISED FOR YEARS.

Take it easy. Often new exercisers find that their heart and lungs rise to the challenge quicker than the skeleton and muscles. Result: they get injured (and give up).

When you start over, the only thing you really need to focus on is not getting injured. Warm up properly, build up slowly and don't do more today than you will be able to do tomorrow.

So start with a nice walk.

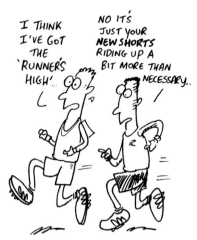

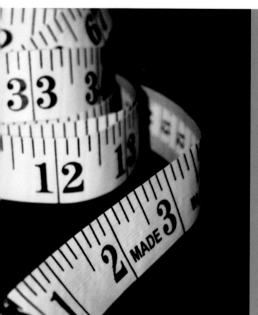

NEED TO LOSE WEIGHT?

Being overweight increases your risk of heart disease, stroke, diabetes and some types of cancer.

Next year in England and Wales alone around 50,000 deaths will be down to excess weight.

So get the tape measure out. As a man, you have a:

> **HIGHER** risk of health problems if your waist size is more than 94cm (37 inches) and an

> **EVEN HIGHER** risk if your waist size is more than 102cm (40 inches.)

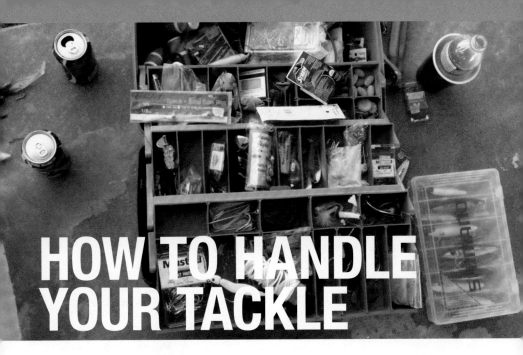

HOW TO HANDLE YOUR TACKLE

We get asked more questions about the male tackle than anything else. This is what men usually want to know.

IS MY PENIS TOO SMALL?

Limp penises come in all shapes and sizes but erect, they're pretty much the same. Not that it matters: the vagina can expand or contract to take anything from a tampon to a baby.

Genuine problems that might stop you enjoying sex or taking a piss are rare and usually picked up when you're a baby. If you've passed that stage, you're probably good to go.

Trying to enlarge your penis is expensive, probably dangerous and almost certainly won't work. Don't. All surgery has risks. You only have one knob and it cannot be replaced.

> Saw my GP. Got my sex life back. It was that simple.

CAN I ASK ABOUT MASTURBATION?

You can and it's fine. Ejaculation is a need like food and drink. It may also reduce the risk of prostate cancer or a tight foreskin. Three health warnings:

> You only have one penis so be careful what you stick it in.

> Anything pleasurable can be addictive.

> Porn is unrealistic, makes human beings into sexual objects and can spoil real relationships with real people.

I COME TOO QUICKLY

Premature ejaculation (PE) is very common. It's usually caused by stress or anxiety. It can nearly always be treated. There are techniques to try yourself - see the Men's Health Forum website - or your GP can prescribe.

I CAN'T GET AN ERECTION

Erectile dysfunction (ED) affects most men at some time (about 1 in 10 of us at any given moment). Often the cause is physical:

> diabetes

> blocked arteries (see page 6 on the heart)

> drinking too much

> drug side-effects

> spinal cord injury

> prostate or other surgery in this area.

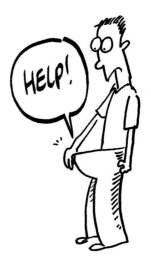

But if you can't get an erection with your partner but can when masturbating or during the night, there's a good chance your ED has psychological causes:

> relationship problems or sexual boredom

> tiredness, stress, depression or anxiety

> sexual identity problem.

You can buy ED drugs in a pharmacy now. That's good. But it's still best to talk to the pharmacist or a GP beforehand. That's because life-threatening problems like heart disease and diabetes can cause ED and you need a professional to rule these out.

MY ERECTION IS BENT

Some bend is normal but if it's so bent that it makes sex uncomfortable, it could be a condition called Peyronie's. Ask your GP about it.

MY ERECTION WON'T GO DOWN

An erection that lasts more than four hours could be a condition called priapism. See a doctor right away. Untreated priapism can be dangerous leading to, for example, permanent erection problems.

MY PENIS IS SORE, RED OR ITCHY

A red, sore penis head could be balanitis. This occurs in uncircumcised men who don't wash their dicks. Your GP can treat it and advise on prevention.

If you've had unprotected sex, it may be a sexually-transmitted infection (STI).

COULD I HAVE AN STI?

Sexually-transmitted infections (STIs) can be caught through vaginal, oral or anal sex. Or skin-to-skin contact. Some STIs are increasing rapidly. Common symptoms include:

> a yellow discharge from your penis

> swollen tender testicles

> irritation of your penis

> pain when peeing.

Your GP can help. Or for something more anonymous, try a specialist sexual health clinic. Many STIs can be treated if caught early, usually with antibiotics.

> I like condoms now I use them properly. You last longer.

Some STIs such as chlamydia may not have any symptoms while the only signs of HIV or hepatitis may be a short flu-like illness. All are serious diseases. So get yourself tested if you've had unsafe sex. The best way to avoid an STI is through safer sex.

WHAT'S SAFER SEX?

Assuming you don't want to stop sex with other people altogether, it's about using condoms. These prevent pregnancy and help prevent most STIs.

Other forms of contraception - like the pill - may stop pregnancy but not STIs. So it's as simple as this: if you don't know someone else's sexual history, use a condom - whatever sort of sex you're having.

> There's more on sex and health for gay men in the Forum's manual Man To Man.

If a condom breaks, the NHS website can direct you to the nearest emergency contraception service.

THERE'S BLOOD IN MY SEMEN/URINE

It's probably nothing but could be a symptom of something more serious like a prostate problem so see your GP. For semen, go if you get blood twice. For urine, once.

MY FORESKIN IS TIGHT. DO I NEED CIRCUMCISION?

Probably not. Frequent, careful, lubricated masturbation can help. (Honest.) Your GP can also advise on creams and stretching techniques. A last resort is full or partial circumcision but that comes with risks.

THE HOLE IN MY PENIS IS IN THE WRONG PLACE

If you're not pissing out of the end of your penis you may have undiagnosed hypospadias. It can be treated, improving both peeing and sexual function. Your GP can refer you to a urology specialist.

I'VE LOST INTEREST IN SEX

Your interest in sex (libido) is a complicated mix of emotions and hormones. Ups and downs with time and age are normal. Libido can also be reduced by:

SORRY TO HAVE TO BREAK THIS TO YOU MATE BUT WEARING EXTRA STRONG DEODORANT DURING SEX ISN'T COUNTED AS 'PROTECTION'...

> tiredness, stress, depression and/or relationship problems

> the side-effects of drink or drugs (including legal drugs such as anti-depressants and blood pressure medication)

> hormonal changes (as men age, levels of testosterone go down)

> medical conditions such as heart disease or diabetes.

If prolonged loss of libido concerns you, see your GP.

I HAVE PAIN/A LUMP IN MY TESTICLES

Testicular cancer is the most common cancer in younger men but remains rare. If you notice a lump in your balls, see your GP immediately. Testicular cancer can be treated very successfully if caught early on.

CAN YOU GET PENIS CANCER?

Yes. But it's very rare. If you have a lump or sore, see your GP or sexual health clinic.

SHOULD I HAVE A VASECTOMY?

If you are sure you want no more children, a vasectomy is a 99.8% effective solution to unwanted pregnancy.

But used properly, condoms are 98% effective. No surgery is without risk and some men - perhaps 10% - have pain and other problems after vasectomies. Remember too that some men change their mind once in a new relationship and vasectomy reversal isn't always successful.

Get advice and think it through.

TELL ME ABOUT THE PROSTATE

The prostate is a small gland producing the thick, white fluid that gets mixed with sperm to create semen. It sits right next to the bladder. As we get older, it is common for the prostate to grow, pushing on the bladder and causing peeing problems.

All of these could be the sign of a prostate problem:

> a weak flow when peeing

> a flow which stops and starts

> having to wait before you start to go

> having to pee more often than previously

> a sudden urgent need to pee

> peeing more often at night.

An enlarged prostate doesn't mean cancer. Often growth is benign. But you need to see your GP to check and get advice on the various treatments.

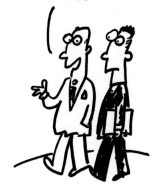

Incontinence (peeing when you don't want to) may also be a sign of prostate growth but there are other causes too. See your GP.

DON'T PUT OFF GOING TO THE GP UNTIL YOU CAN'T PEE AT ALL

I play golf and usually need a pee during a round. But I was finding it wasn't so easy. I was dashing into the woods two or three times. It took ages to start and I was having to stop to catch the lads up.

After say four years, I saw my GP. I was told I had a very enlarged prostate but no sign of cancer. So I left it another year. One day, I had a long meeting and left it too long. When I finally went to pee, I was desperate but couldn't go at all. It was awful. The internet told me it was acute retention and to get to the doctor immediately.

Fifteen minutes later, the doctor was fitting a catheter in my penis. I'd been healthy all my life and suddenly a woman was sticking a plastic tube up my willy so as to empty my bladder. It was traumatic. It's not even embarrassing because you're in so much pain, you just want something done. The relief as you finally feel the bladder begin to empty is enormous despite the catheter pain.

The catheter came out after two weeks but I had acute retention again. This time they couldn't get the catheter in. It was so painful. I had to go to the hospital which was 45 minutes away.

I knew this wasn't going to solve itself with drugs. I'd been put on alpha-blockers which are the usual treatment but had side-effects like headaches and dizziness. I knew I needed a surgical solution. I looked at several but didn't like the idea of lasers and the possible retrograde ejaculation and erection problems. In the end I chose the prostate arterial embolisation (PAE). This blocks some of the blood supply to the prostate preventing growth.

Today, I don't pee like I did when I was 19 but the PAE has rolled back the clock 20 years. I would say to anyone with peeing problems, see your GP. It is going to get worse and finish in acute retention unless you do something. I was in denial. I hoped the problem would go away or not get worse. The actual PAE hardly inconvenienced me at all but the acute retention was the worst.

PAE is one of a number of less-invasive treatments now becoming available for enlarged prostates.

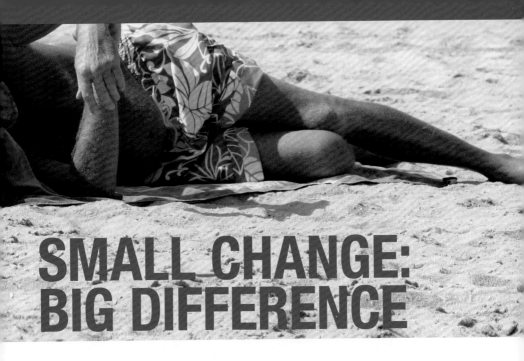

SMALL CHANGE: BIG DIFFERENCE

Most of us want to make little changes which will make our lives more fun. For example, most smokers want to quit.

HOW DO I QUIT SMOKING?

We all know ciggies are bad for our health. Less well known is how quickly you start to feel better after quitting. Here are some tips to help:

> List all your reasons for quitting.

> Set the day in advance (when doing something new can be a good time such as going on holiday or starting a new job).

> Get rid of all your smoking stuff at home, work, in the car etc.

> Team up with a friend or two to quit together.

> Try to avoid smokers.

> Try to avoid places or circumstances in which you usually smoke.

> When you get a craving, talk to someone, go for a walk, drink water or nibble on a healthy snack (carrots are good), get a change of scene or do something that will keep you busy.

> Take it a day at a time and mark your progress.

> Put the money you save to one side and watch it grow.

> Don't be tempted to have 'just one' - it doesn't work.

I saved £1500 in six months. It paid for a great holiday.

> Check out NHS Smokefree online. They can direct you to local Stop Smoking services and other stuff to help you quit. Download their app.

> I got very very badly sunburnt in just half an hour.

ARE E-CIGARETTES OK?

If you used to smoke and now vape, e-cigarettes may be a step in the right direction. But watch out: you're still addicted to nicotine and the step between smoking and not smoking is smaller when you vape meaning it's easier to slip back into the tobacco habit or fall into it for the first time. Research continues on the effects of vaping. But e-cigarettes are not just hot air - they are a regulated product.

AM I ADDICTED?

You can have too much of a good thing. Think you might be addicted to drink, drugs, gambling, gaming, porn or something else? Even work, exercise or your phone. Ask yourself these questions:

> Do you think about X while doing something else and look forward to it?

> Do you feel you need more X each time to get the same enjoyment?

> Have you made efforts to cut back on X?

> Do you do X for longer than intended?

> Have you put X before more important things like relationships or work?

> Have you lied to others about your involvement with X?

> Do you use X as a way of escaping from problems or of relieving, for example, feelings of guilt, anxiety or depression?

If the answer to any of these is yes, you need to stop doing X. If you can't stop, you need to talk to someone. It's that simple.

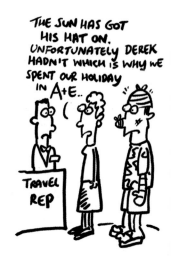

THE SUN HAS GOT HIS HAT ON. UNFORTUNATELY DEREK HADN'T WHICH IS WHY WE SPENT OUR HOLIDAY IN A+E..

TRAVEL REP

You're not alone - at least two million people in the UK are fighting an addiction. There's no shame. Some men are tall. Some get colds. Some get addicted. The problems really begin if you can't admit the truth to yourself. Talk to a mate, family member, your GP or an organisation working with people with the same challenge as you.

HOW DANGEROUS IS THE SUN?

It can be very dangerous. The number of people in hospital for skin cancer is increasing. What's more, men are more likely to die from the disease than women. The main cause of skin cancer is the sun. If you have fair skin, light-coloured eyes or more moles, you're at higher risk.

Don't avoid the sun. Being outside is good for you. But cover up. Wear a shirt and hat. Choose sunscreen that is at least SPF 15+ and has a **** rating.

Keep an eye on your moles. You're looking for changes to the ABCDE:

A – asymmetry (both halves should look the same)

B – border irregularity (it should be round)

C – colour change (it should be tan - not red, black or white)

D – diameter (it should be below 4mm)

E – elevated (raised) or enlarged.

Also watch for itchiness or bleeding. Any concerns, see your GP.

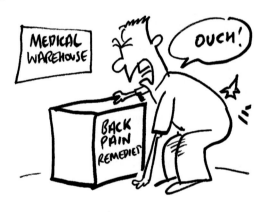

HOW DO I PROTECT MY BACK?

Back pain is a major cause of lost working days and on the increase as we live longer. In the UK, four out of five of us are affected at some time in our lives.

The key thing is to keep active. Immobility weakens muscles and reduces range of movement.

Think about your back when staying in the same position for some time.

Lift with a straight back and with the load close to your waist. Distribute weight evenly and know your limits.

Exercise will both prevent and reduce back pain. Find out about exercises to strengthen your 'core' (muscles in your abdomen, back and around the the pelvis). Try yoga or pilates. If you're overweight, lose some. Over-the-counter painkillers may help in the short term but if back pain persists, see your GP.

I USE TECHNOLOGY ALL THE TIME. ANY WORRIES?

Staying in the same position for too long, especially unnatural positions like on the train or on the couch, may affect your back. The screen may affect your eyes. Look away, take screen breaks and get up regularly to move around. Can you stand to work rather than sitting all the time?

At your desk, note how you're sitting, the computer screen position, your chair height, the position of your mouse and keyboard and the rest of your desk equipment. Adjust your position so your eyes are level with the screen, arms are comfortable and supported and the chair supports your back. If using a laptop for a long period, try a separate keyboard and mouse and a laptop stand. (Remember too that using a laptop actually on your lap can damage sperm and fertility.)

It makes sense to turn devices off sometimes not least because of the proven high health risk from using them when distraction can be dangerous. For example, using a handheld phone while driving is illegal and hands-free is not advised. But there's also the fact that too much time on your screen can mean less time for real relationships with real people.

SHOULD I GET MY SIGHT TESTED?

See an optometrist if you are having difficulty focusing close up or seeing long distance or have pain, headaches, blurred vision or see halos around lights. As we age, some deterioration in sight is normal. The basic eye test is cheaper than you think and is free in many cases or if 'clinically necessary'.

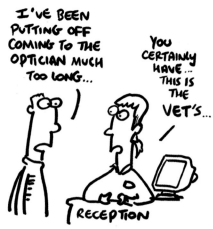

If you already wear glasses or contacts, you should go for an eye test at least every couple of years. People over 40 and people from black or minority ethnic groups may need tests more frequently. (People from African-Caribbean backgrounds are at greater risk of glaucoma and diabetes and people from south Asian backgrounds at greater risk of diabetes.)

If you use screens habitually as a significant part of your normal work, your employer should pay for a proper eye test and any glasses you might need for screen work.

Always protect eyes when working by using the right mask, shield or goggles.

WHAT ABOUT HEARING?

Hearing also deteriorates with age - 40% of those over 50 have some hearing loss. Look after your ears by wearing ear protectors when necessary and keeping volume down when using headphones or headsets.

Wax build-up can also affect hearing. Warmed olive oil (yes, the cooking type) can loosen wax, or try drops from your pharmacist. If they don't help, see your practice nurse.

DO I HAVE TO GO TO THE DENTIST?

Yes - at least once a year. It could prevent a lot of pain and expense later on.

You can reduce the risk considerably by brushing twice a day for two minutes at a time with toothpaste. (The NHS suggests fluoride toothpaste.) Brush all surfaces including the gums gently with an up-and-down motion. Flossing or interdental brushes can help you clean between the teeth.

Cleaning gets rid of the bacteria (plaque) that cause tooth decay and gum disease.

Mouth cancer is more common in men than women. Watch out for white or red patches, ulcers or lumps that do not clear up after two weeks, especially if you smoke and drink.

DO YOU KNOW YOUR FAMILY HISTORY?

Many health problems run in families: heart disease, cancer, strokes, depression, mental health challenges.

Find out if your parents, grandparents, aunts and uncles have had any of these illnesses, especially if they died young.

Make sure your GP knows your family health history.

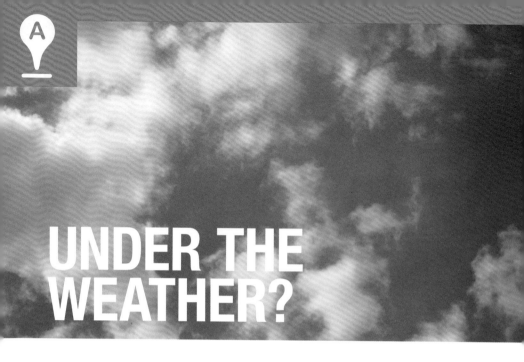

UNDER THE WEATHER?

WHAT SHOULD I DO WHEN I'M ILL?

For coughs, colds, other minor problems and advice on treatment and local services, try your high-street pharmacist. There's one on most high streets. Just walk in. Many have a private area to talk if need be.

For illness or personalised advice, the local general practice (GP) is the first point of contact. Make sure you're registered with one. It's very easy to do. Choose one that is easy to get to from home or work. Check opening hours, the appointment system and what you can do online or by phone.

General practices also provide information, vaccinations, clinics, health-checks, blood tests and some simple operations.

Call 111 if you need advice but it's not a life-threatening situation. 111 is also online at 111.nhs.uk. (111 can also tell you which NHS service you need.)

WHAT ABOUT OUT OF HOURS?

Out of hours, contact 111 or your GP's out-of-hours service.

In an emergency, call 999 or go to a hospital Accident and Emergency Department (A&E).

My complex diabetes is the direct result of not going to the GP.

WHAT'S AN EMERGENCY?

Call 999 or go to A&E if the patient is:

> unconscious

> in a very confused state

> having fits that are not stopping

> having breathing difficulties

> having persistent, severe chest pain

> bleeding severely and you cannot stop it.

You are wasting your time and everybody else's if you go to A&E and it is not an emergency.

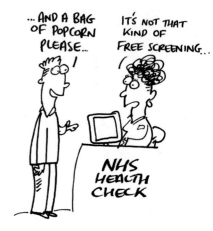

> The A&E staff were great. The four-hour wait wasn't.

... AND A BAG OF POPCORN PLEASE...

IT'S NOT THAT KIND OF FREE SCREENING...

NHS HEALTH CHECK

MY GP IS TOO BUSY.

The NHS is overstretched. You will get the best out of it if you make things as easy as you can for your GP (or any other health professional you see).

Turn up in good time. Note the questions you want answered. Answer their questions honestly.

Get to the point - don't save what's really on your mind until you're about to leave. Make sure you understand what's going on with any treatment or drugs prescribed before you leave.

Take advantage of the service when you get the chance: if you're invited for a health check or screening, go along.

WHAT OTHER NHS SERVICES ARE THERE?

There are specific NHS services for, for example, stopping smoking or mental health problems. Sexual health clinics offer free confidential advice, testing and treatment for sexually-transmitted infections.

The NHS also has a mix of walk-in centres, urgent care centres, minor injury units and urgent treatment centres, each offering different services. They may be quicker and easier for non-emergency injuries like sprains, breaks, minor burns and bites.

These are generally called urgent treatment centres. They should be led by GPs and open for at least 12 hours a day every day of the week.

You can find services near you on the Men's Health Forum or NHS websites.

WHAT ABOUT THE INTERNET?

When searching be aware of who runs the sites you're visiting. Look for sites that display the NHS England Information Standard 'Health and care information you can trust' logo. (You can see the logo on page 2.) Be sceptical of social media and commercial sites without this. On overseas sites, the HONcode is a sign of quality.

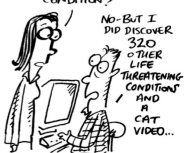

When researching online, be honest with yourself about what you do and don't know about health. We tend to think the web and socal media make us an expert in everything. They don't. The web can be a valuable tool but it is also full of misinformation. Many people misdiagnose themselves.

The Men's Health Forum or NHS websites provide lots of useful information. But information is all it is. You need a doctor to diagnose.

IS IT OK TO BUY DRUGS ONLINE?

If you have a prescription from a GP, many GPs and pharmacists can deal with these online.

If you don't have a prescription, get one. Don't self-diagnose and buy drugs online. Many sites offering drugs without prescription are illegal. The drugs they sell may be useless or dangerous fakes. Plus your credit card details may be stolen.

> I paid £130 for a product that didn't work.

Perhaps even more importantly, you won't get a diagnosis of your problem. Not being able to get an erection won't kill you. But heart disease or diabetes (of which erection problems are a sign) can.